CHRIS HAYHURST

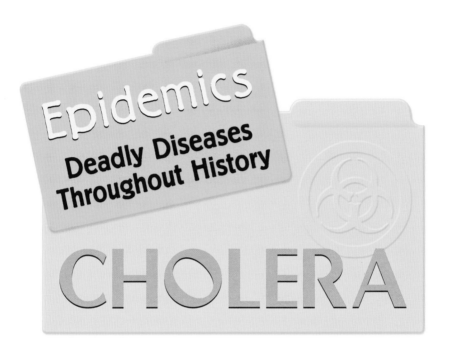

Epidemics
Deadly Diseases
Throughout History

CHOLERA

The Rosen Publishing Group, Inc.
New York

Published in 2001 by The Rosen Publishing Group, Inc.
29 East 21st Street, New York, NY 10010

Copyright © 2001 by The Rosen Publishing Group, Inc.

First Edition

Library of Congress Cataloging-in-Publication Data

Hayhurst, Chris.
    Cholera / by Chris Hayhurst. — 1st ed.
        p.   cm. — (Epidemics!)
Includes bibliographical references and index.
    ISBN 0-8239-3345-8 (lib. bdg.)
    1. Cholera—Juvenile literature. [1. Cholera. 2. Diseases.]
I. Title. II. Series.
    RC126 .H43 2000
    616.9'32—dc21

                                                    00-009905

Cover image: *Vibrio* cholera.

Manufactured in the United States of America

CONTENTS

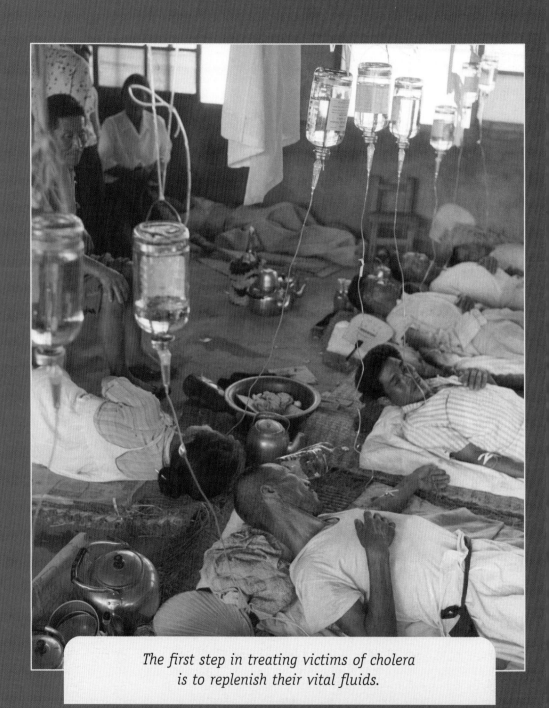

*The first step in treating victims of cholera
is to replenish their vital fluids.*

INTRODUCTION

The year was 1854. The place, London, England. It was summer. And in one very unlucky neighborhood—a rather busy part of town known as Broad Street, Golden Square—people were dying everywhere.

Diarrhea poured like water from the withering bodies of the sick. Intense vomiting sent people to their knees, hunched over in agony, tears streaming from their eyes. Paralyzing muscle cramps tied victims in knots. Some died in their sleep. Others suffered in hospital beds. Children, playing in the streets one minute, lay sprawled on the ground only hours later.

Many individuals and families fled the area in fear and desperation, leaving their belongings behind. The situation seemed hopeless. More

1817
First reported cholera epidemic takes place in India.

Early 1830s
John Snow, an epidemiologist—a scientist who studies how diseases occur and spread in populations—begins studying cholera by working with patients who are infected with the disease.

1849
Snow develops theory that cholera is a water-borne disease.

1849
Cholera outbreak takes place in Chicago and 678 people die.

than 500 people died in just ten days. The reason? A disease called cholera.

Cholera, while not well understood, was not new to the world during that deadly summer season less than 150 years ago. In fact, in India, where the disease is believed to have originated, ancient writings described strikingly similar catastrophes more than 2,000 years earlier. More recently, in 1817, the disease had hammered India again and gone on to spread around much of the globe. London, and the Broad Street neighborhood in particular, was just one stop along the disease's devastating path of destruction—a path which continues even today.

1854
Cholera breaks out in London, England.

1854
In London, Snow presents and tests theory about cholera being a water-borne disease. Tests are a success.

1855
Snow publishes *On the Mode of Cholera*, which spells out his theory.

1947
Cholera breaks out in Egypt.

(continued)

Still, if the outbreak on Broad Street wasn't a complete surprise, it was noteworthy for one major reason. It was there, in a neighborhood of just a few blocks, that the key to understanding cholera—what it is, what causes it, and how it can be prevented and cured—was finally turned. This maddening and mysterious disease that had killed millions and would, over time, kill millions more, was about to be poked, prodded, examined, and, ultimately, explained. People might die, but soon, at least, they'd know why.

Today cholera is no mystery. Scientists and doctors have examined the disease thoroughly. They know that it's caused by a nasty bacterium—a microscopic

1961
Worldwide cholera pandemic begins on Indonesian island of Celebes.

1964
Pandemic hits India.

1970
Pandemic hits South Africa.

1963
Pandemic hits Bangladesh.

1965
Pandemic hits Soviet Union.

organism consisting of just one tiny cell—called *Vibrio cholerae*. And they also know exactly how this bacterium is spread.

People usually contract cholera when they drink water or eat food that is contaminated with *Vibrio cholerae*. The tiny bacteria hitch a ride, on the food or in the drink, into a person's small intestine, where digested nutrients are normally absorbed into the body. This is where the trouble starts. Within a day or two, if all goes well for the *Vibrio cholerae*, an infection develops along the walls of the intestine. A chemical reaction takes place. Often the infection is

1973
Pandemic hits Europe.

1991
Pandemic hits South America.

1992
New strain of cholera breaks out in India and Bangladesh.

1981
Seventeen people contract cholera on an oil rig off the coast of Texas.

1991
Eight cases of cholera reported in New Jersey.

rather tame and the person shows no symptoms of the disease. He or she just goes on eating and drinking and living life the same way. Sometimes, however, things get bad—fast.

The first sign of cholera is a severe case of watery diarrhea. Then comes vomiting. In the worst cases, the diarrhea is so terrible it literally gushes from the body like water. In fact, for the most part, it is water. And therein lies the next problem: dehydration. As the victim loses body fluids, he or she becomes severely dehydrated. When left untreated, dehydration can be extremely dangerous. Leg muscles cramp.

Some people think the word "cholera" may have originated from the Greek word for "roof gutter"—picture rainwater gushing from a gutter following a major drenching and it's easy to imagine why.

The skin becomes cold and droops. The circulatory system, which keeps blood flowing to all parts of the body, may collapse. Blood pressure drops. The victim may go into shock, a life-threatening condition that occurs when not enough blood makes it to the head. Kidneys and other major organs may shut down. Death is possible in just a few hours if nothing is done.

Of course, today, with the help of modern medicine and well-trained doctors, something is usually done. In fact, the disease can be treated quite easily. All a victim needs to do is keep from becoming dehydrated. According to the Centers for Disease Control (CDC), a governmental organization in the United States that combats many different diseases, fewer than 1 percent of cholera victims die if they get the fluids they need right away. The first goal of a doctor treating a cholera victim is to replenish the vital salts and fluids the victim has lost through diarrhea and vomiting. This is often done by getting the victim to drink water and sip liquid foods such as soup. But sometimes that's not as easy as it sounds. If you're extremely sick and throwing up, it can be almost impossible to drink or eat.

"Usually the patient is moribund (approaching death), eyes sunken back into the skull, literally minutes away from death. It may be a small child, or a mother, or an elderly man. Then comes the struggle to find a vein, and the first anxious moments as the IV drip starts to run. Always then I must move on to the next bed, and I may not have time to come back until many hours later. By then the patient has come back to life—sitting up, drinking, even managing a smile. It is the nearest thing to a miracle that a doctor ever gets to perform."

—Medécins sans Frontières field doctor, Bangladesh. Medécins sans Frontières (Doctors without Borders) is an international humanitarian aid organization that provides medical help to people who need it in more than eighty countries around the world.

To get around this problem, medical practitioners replenish bodily fluids intravenously—by using a needle to inject a special salt-and-water solution directly into the victim's veins. Antibiotics, or drugs designed to destroy the *Vibrio cholerae* bacterium, can also help to make the symptoms less severe.

London Under Siege

A map, made in 1854 by John Snow and published in his book, *On the Mode of Cholera*, showed where victims of the Broad Street cholera outbreak died and was used to understand the spread of the disease. Today, mapping "medical geography," as it's now known, is used all the time by scientists, doctors, and other medical professionals as they strive to learn more about how diseases such as cholera move within a population. Of course, modern-day researchers have much more sophisticated techniques at their disposal than did Snow, who probably did everything by hand. Thanks to computers, special software programs, satellites, and other high-tech gadgets, mapping is now a highly specialized science.

1

THE BIRTH OF A DEADLY DISEASE

Most scientists believe the first major cholera outbreak, or epidemic, took place in eastern India in 1817. Here, in a region known as Bengal, where the Indian Ocean meets the coastline, life was rough. Villagers were poor. Many were starving and undernourished, as drought left much of the land cracked and useless and made it difficult to grow food crops. What water people could scrounge up was dirty, often contaminated with garbage and human sewage.

Looking back, any medical professional could tell you that cholera was bound to break out in this very vulnerable population. The *Vibrio cholerae* bacterium thrives in human feces. And in the unsanitary conditions of early nineteenth-century India, cholera found a welcoming home as feces made it into the water supply and ultimately into the guts of those who drank the water or washed their food in it.

The first cholera epidemic in India lasted for just four years. Still, thousands, even millions, died from the disease. And after the first epidemic came to an end, new ones began. Conditions were ripe. As the sick and hungry sought help, they crowded into relief camps, towns, and cities, spreading cholera as they went. Cholera became a part of life—and a common way to die. People had no clue how to fight the disease effectively. Experts estimate that at least 15 million people died of cholera in India in the first fifty years after that initial outbreak.

Soon after the epidemics in India began, the disease began to travel around the world. Cholera became pandemic, spreading throughout Asia, popping up in Russia, entering Europe, and eventually hitting the Americas. Millions more people died. Because of tremendous developments in worldwide trade and transportation, it was easier for people to travel from one end of the planet to the other. And wherever people traveled, cholera went with them. Contaminated food could be shipped with relative ease from an isolated village in the middle of nowhere to a major city swarming with people. Transportation and technology were revolutionized, making the

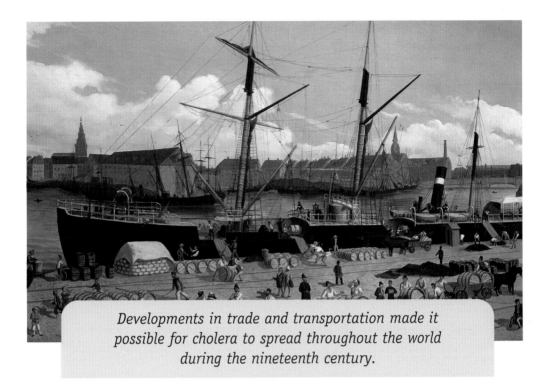

Developments in trade and transportation made it possible for cholera to spread throughout the world during the nineteenth century.

planet more interconnected. But medicine and public health were unable to keep up with the consequences of greater globalization.

For the rest of the nineteenth century, pandemic cholera came and went in waves. Just when people thought the disease had disappeared for good, it would appear again. All told, there were six pandemics between the first outbreak in 1817 and the end of the century. Then, in the first half of the twentieth century, the disease seemed to rest. It was still present in Asia, but aside from a devastating epidemic in Egypt in 1947, it didn't appear in epidemic proportions anywhere else in the world.

Modern Outbreak

Then, in 1961, the world's seventh cholera pandemic kicked in. It was born as an epidemic on the Indonesian island of Celebes and began to spread. Known as *Vibrio cholerae* 01, biotype El Tor, it hit Bangladesh in 1963, India a year later, and the Soviet Union, Iran, and Iraq the year after that. By 1970, El Tor had hit West Africa, a region that hadn't seen cholera for at least a century. From there the disease marched east to engulf the entire African continent.

In 1973 the cholera pandemic spread to Europe. Later that decade it hit Japan and the South Pacific. Still, for those in the Western Hemisphere, including people living in North, South, and Central America, the disease was still relatively unknown. For example, South America hadn't had a cholera outbreak all century.

Good luck never lasts forever, of course, and in January of 1991 cholera swept ashore on the banks of South America. Peru was the first country to be hit. From there, it spread. Fast. Within two years, more than 50 percent of all cholera cases were occurring in the Western Hemisphere. By 1994 almost a million cases of cholera caused by the El Tor biotype had been reported to the World Health Organization (WHO) by twenty-one Western countries.

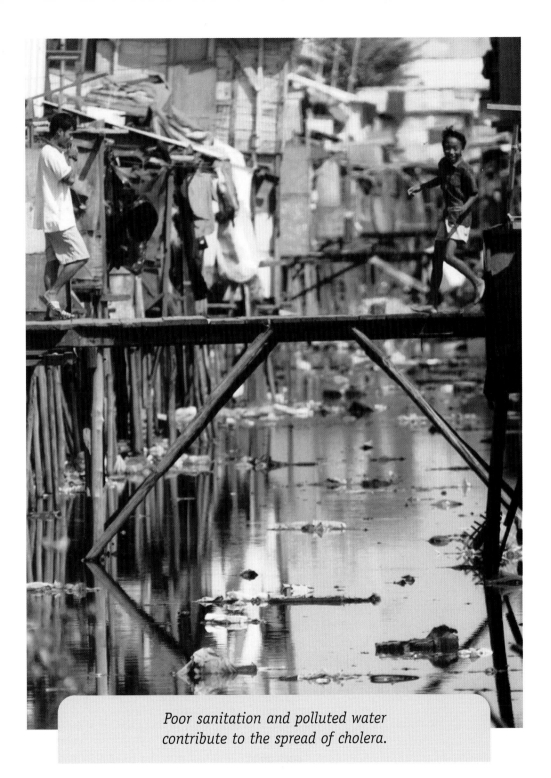

Poor sanitation and polluted water contribute to the spread of cholera.

Today, as the seventh pandemic continues, more than sixty countries report outbreaks to the WHO every year. The disease is all over the world—West Africa, Central America, India, and elsewhere. No one knows when the pandemic will end. All that is known for sure is that as long as poor countries lack proper sanitation and health facilities—and as long as water supplies remain polluted with sewage—cholera will continue to plague those unlucky enough to be caught in its gut-wrenching grip.

2

LESS FAMOUS OUTBREAKS

Not every cholera outbreak becomes as famous as the one in India in 1817 or the episode in London in 1854. Sometimes just one or two people contract the disease while hundreds or thousands of their neighbors remain healthy. Such cases attract very little attention. Sometimes the disease is minor and is not even recognized by doctors for what it is. The victims manage to recover without ever knowing it was cholera that caused their illness.

Here in the United States, cholera has had a very short and relatively quiet history. It pops up once in a while, but never to the extent that it's seen in Africa, Asia, and Latin America. Thanks to well-developed waste-treatment systems and good sanitary conditions in most parts of the United States, cholera almost never has the opportunity to infect people.

Still, when cholera does appear, it definitely turns heads. And such was the case in 1991 in New Jersey. Between March 31st and April 3rd of that year, eight residents of the state became ill after eating crab meat flown in from Ecuador, a country in South America. One of the victims had bought the meat at an Ecuadorian fish market, carried it home on a plane, and served it in a salad to family and friends. Within days of the meal, everyone who ate the meat came down with watery diarrhea. Five of the people experienced vomiting, and three had terrible leg cramps. Five people wound up in the hospital. Doctors who treated the victims examined their stools and found half of them to be contaminated with the El Tor variety of *Vibrio cholerae* 01, the same serotype, or strain, responsible for the January epidemic in South America. Fortunately for all those involved, and thanks to prompt treatment with modern medicine, no one died.

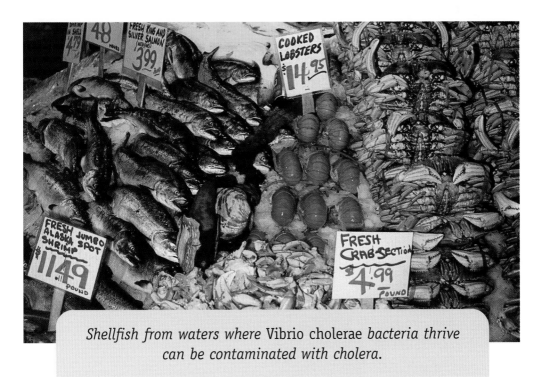

Shellfish from waters where Vibrio cholerae *bacteria thrive can be contaminated with cholera.*

The outbreak in New Jersey wasn't the first time this century that cholera hit the United States. In fact, El Tor had popped up around the country every once in a while for almost twenty years. For example, in 1973 one person contracted cholera in Texas. No one knows why. Five years later there were eight more cases in Louisiana. Later, in 1981, seventeen people came down with the disease while working on a floating oil rig off the coast of Texas. Scientists don't think these cases had anything to do with poor sanitation. Rather, they believe the cholera was contracted when the victims ate shellfish from coastal waters where the *Vibrio cholerae* bacteria thrived. They believe the shellfish were contaminated with cholera and that by eating this fish the people became sick.

Since the 1970s, cholera cases continue to be reported in the United States. Relative to countries in other parts of the world, however, the cases are rare

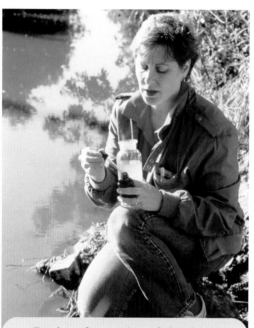

Testing the purity of drinking water is vital in preventing the spread of cholera.

and usually minor. Still, as long as the current epidemic in Latin America rages on, it's likely that people in the United States will, on occasion, contract the disease. All it takes is forgetting to wash a contaminated fruit or vegetable, or drinking water that is contaminated. Experts aren't sure how long the epidemic will last, but they do agree that progress can only be made if sanitation measures in Latin American countries are improved.

Once sewage and water-treatment systems are brought up to standard, future cholera outbreaks will become far less likely.

Cholera hit Chicago several times in the 1800s. Experts believe the city's first bout with the disease, in 1849, took place when immigrants unknowingly brought it with them to the United States from overseas. That year was devastating to the city—678 people died. In the following years, Chicago did a number of things to improve the quality of its drinking water and sewage systems, and by the 1870s cholera was no longer a problem.

YEAR	DEATHS IN CHICAGO
1849	678
1850	420
1851	216
1852	630
1853	1
1854	1,424
1855	147
1856–1865	not significant
1866	990
1867	10

Source: Chicago Public Library

A New Strain

Until relatively recently, *Vibrio cholerae* 01 was the only serotype of the bacteria known to cause epidemic cholera. Other serotypes were well known to scientists, but they never caused more than basic diarrhea, and certainly never led to anything of epidemic proportions.

That changed in 1992 when large outbreaks in India and Bangladesh were caused by a previously unknown serotype that scientists designated "0139," or "Bengal." Since the discovery of this new strain, it has appeared in almost a dozen Asian countries. Will it spread even further, to other regions and other parts of the world? Will it become pandemic? For now, say scientists, there's no way of knowing. Meanwhile, they're doing everything they can to learn more about this strain, predict where it might show up next, and figure out how it can be contained.

3

SCIENCE

Scientists know a lot about cholera. They know how it enters the human body and how it exits. They know that it's spread by contaminated food and water supplies, and therefore tends to be most common in poor parts of the world where sanitation is not adequate.

One of the most interesting things about cholera is how it's spread from region to region—not just from one person to the next, but from one continent to another. Scientists now know, for example, that both human actions and natural environmental occurrences, like climate changes, contribute to the spread of deadly microbes like the *Vibrio cholerae* bacteria.

Some scientists have noted that the 1991 cholera outbreak in Latin America may have

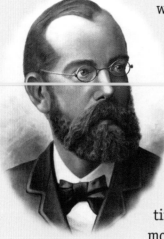

Robert Koch

Every once in a while a person is born who makes a real difference in how the world works. Robert Koch, a scientist born in Clausthal, Germany, in 1843, was one of those people. Koch was one of the founders of the science of bacteriology (the study of bacteria) and showed that specific microorganisms, or bacteria, cause specific diseases.

Working in the late 1800s, at a time when cholera was one of the most feared and deadly diseases in the world, Koch spent many long hours in his laboratory and traveled the world. He had a problem, though. While he and other scientists had an idea that microscopic organisms were behind diseases like cholera, no one had been able to prove that these microbes even existed. In fact, they were impossible to see, even through a microscope.

Fortunately, Koch came up with a solution. He found a way to stain the microbes with dye. The dye allowed him to photograph the microbes under a microscope and study them more effectively. Using this technique, he was able to identify the microbes that cause tuberculosis in 1882. A year later, in 1883, he determined exactly which bacteria cause cholera and found that the cholera organism can be carried in water and on food.

Koch's work, which included trips to Egypt and India, where cholera was rampant, eventually led to proof that pollution by certain bacteria spread disease. Water polluted with cholera bacteria, for example, spread cholera to those who drank it. His research also showed that the cholera bacteria could spread from population to population through the diarrhea of its victims. By the turn of the century, Koch and his assistants had used the microbe-dyeing method to identify more than twenty specific germs that cause disease. As a result of this work, he won the Nobel Prize for Physiology and Medicine in 1905.

been due at least in part to the warmer temperatures caused by the El Niño weather patterns, which could have created the warm conditions that are ideal for the cholera bacteria. Another factor in the disease's emergence in South America for the first time in decades may have been increased international trade and the ease with which goods (and any microbes they may be carrying) are now shipped throughout the world. It is quite easy for food contaminated with cholera to travel from one end of the world to the other. And finally, Peru had recently reduced certain measures it normally used to ensure that its water supply was pure and bacteria-free, like treatment with chlorine. This may have also aided the emergence of the disease.

Where do you get your drinking water? From a lake? From a stream? From a private well deep beneath the ground? Or do you drink only bottled water? Depending on where you live, you probably drink water that comes from one or more of these sources. But do you have any idea what that water contains?

Probably not. And to be honest, your water is, most likely, perfectly safe to drink. Thanks to the Clean Water Act, which was passed into law by the U.S. Congress in 1972, polluted waterways are relatively rare. Cities are now required to maintain wastewater treatment plants that keep polluted water from entering our drinking-water supplies. States are also required to adhere to strict water-quality standards. Tap water rules prohibit contamination with bacteria like *E. coli* or fecal coliform, which would be present if the water contained fecal matter. In big cities that use surface waters, such as rivers, lakes, or streams, for their drinking-water supply, the Environmental Protection Agency (EPA) requires the use of filtering or disinfectants to prevent contamination of water with cholera bacteria.

In the United States, the likelihood of contracting a disease like cholera by drinking tap water is extremely slim. Still, it never hurts to keep tabs on your water. In the same way you would examine the list of ingredients on a box of cereal, it's a good idea to see exactly what's in the water that pours from your tap.

For more information on drinking-water safety, water pollution, ocean waters, and water conservation, among other issues, contact the Natural Resources Defense Council,

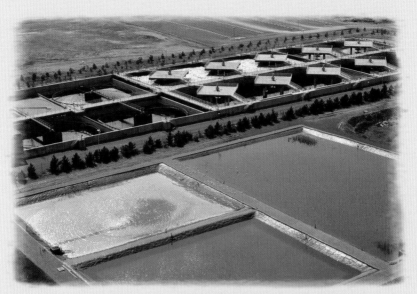

The Clean Water Act of 1972 requires U.S. cities to maintain wastewater treatment plants.

40 West 20th Street, New York, NY 10011; (212) 727-2700; www.nrdc.org. For a list of laboratories certified by your state to test drinking water, as well as basic information about drinking water and the EPA's drinking-water program, call the EPA's Safe Drinking Water Hotline at (800) 426-4791 or go to www.epa.gov/safewater. Alternatively, look up your local, county, or state health departments in the phone book. You'll find them listed under "Health" or "Government." Some local health departments test private water, such as well water, for free. Finally, if you're interested in filtering your tap water yourself, purchase a filter certified by the National Sanitation Foundation (800) NSF-MARK (673-6275).

Other countries have been stricken by cholera thanks to the migration of people. For example, war forces people to flee their homes. Sometimes they end up crowded into refugee camps, where conditions are unsanitary and limited medical supplies are devoted to many problems other than cholera. Economic conditions can also play a part. Poor people from small villages where cholera is endemic may move to cities to look for work and end up bringing the disease with them.

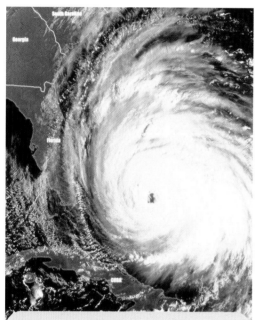

The warm conditions created by the El Niño weather pattern may have contributed to the spread of cholera.

Despite the fact that doctors and other medical experts are well aware of how to prevent cholera outbreaks and how to treat them when they do occur, cholera continues to be a major threat to public health in many parts of the world. When established medical facilities are removed or understaffed, or when cholera strikes a region of the world where such facilities never existed, the disease becomes dangerous

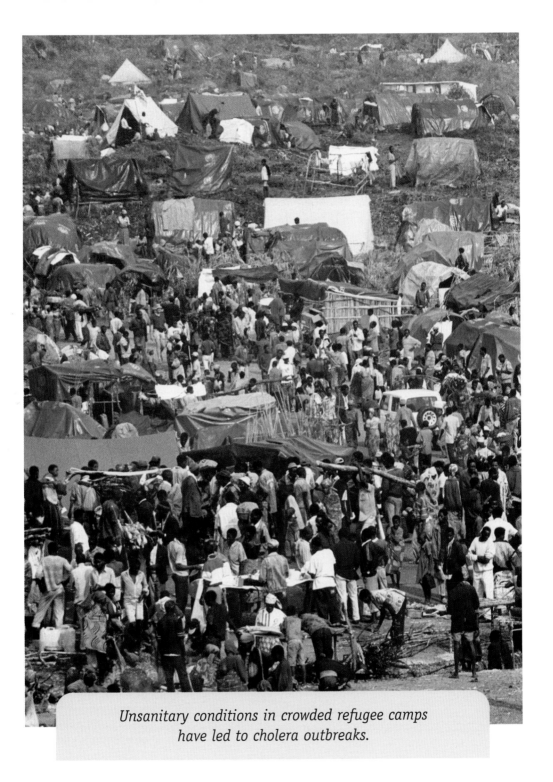

Unsanitary conditions in crowded refugee camps have led to cholera outbreaks.

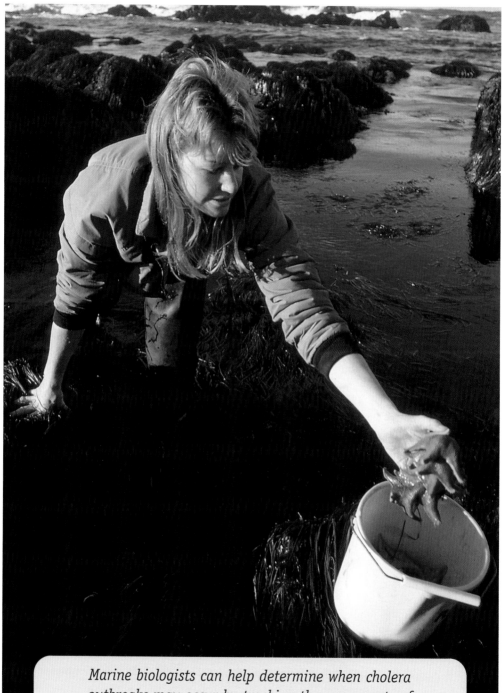

Marine biologists can help determine when cholera outbreaks may occur by tracking the movements of organisms that Vibrio cholerae *bacteria often live on.*

and has the potential to kill many people. Even in the industrialized world, where diseases of epidemic proportions don't often strike, cholera can break out in cities where water purification is not adequate or has been disabled. All over the world, cholera appears in places where public health measures have broken down and reliable water supplies no longer exist.

Tracking Cholera

Since the days of London's Broad Street epidemic in the mid-1800s, technology has changed tremendously. Modern-day scientists now use a number of disciplines, including ecology, oceanography, microbiology, marine biology, and epidemiology, to predict when cholera epidemics are likely to occur. It's even possible to track *Vibrio cholerae* with special space-based satellite imaging equipment designed to follow the movements of ocean organisms that the bacteria often live on. By determining when these marine organisms (and their hitchhiking *Vibrio cholerae* partners) are going to hit shore, scientists can predict when a coastal area is most vulnerable to a cholera outbreak and can warn people to take extra care with their food and water. The technology also gives medical professionals and aid workers time to prepare medicine and facilities for an epidemic before it takes place.

No discussion about epidemiology—the science of how diseases occur and spread in populations—would be complete without mentioning Dr. John Snow. Snow, born in York, England, on March 15, 1813, was the first person to prove that cholera could be carried in water polluted by sewage.

Snow was not an epidemiologist by trade, but a highly respected anesthesiologist. He was one of the first doctors to use drugs such as ether and chloroform to temporarily knock people out or ease their pain during operations.

Snow became interested in cholera in the early 1830s as he worked on patients who were sick from the disease. Back then, no one knew for sure how cholera was spread. Most people believed it was possible to contract the disease just by breathing near someone who was already sick. The theory was that if you inhaled infected air, you stood a good chance of getting cholera.

By 1849, however, Snow had a theory of his own. During his years working on London's cholera victims, he had observed that most deaths from the disease occurred among those who got their water downstream from the city's major sewers. This led him to believe that cholera was contracted not through the air, but by swallowing water contaminated with sewage from other cholera victims. Backing up his theory was the fact that most of London's drinking water was unfiltered and unsanitary.

Proof for Snow's theory finally came in the summer of 1854. It was late August, and an outbreak of cholera had just begun to hit a London neighborhood. Snow, convinced that people were becoming ill because of the water they were drinking, was determined to put an end to the epidemic as soon as possible. Hundreds of people were dying. Thousands more were at risk.

To pinpoint the source of the disease, Snow used a map of the area to plot points showing exactly where each person had died. He also noted the source of the neighborhood's water supply, a pump on Broad Street. Looking at his map, the answer was obvious. Most of the deaths up until that point were clustered within a few hundred yards of the water pump. The people who were dying were the same people who drew their water from the Broad Street pump. Certain he had found the source of the outbreak, Snow went to the pump himself and took a look at the water. Even without a microscope, he could see that the water was filthy. He knew he had found the culprit.

On September 7, 1854, Snow presented his research to the local authorities and asked them to remove the pump's handle to prevent more people from drinking the water. The next day the handle was taken away, and the epidemic was stopped cold in its tracks. Thousands of lives were saved.

The following year, Snow published a book called *On the Mode of Communication of Cholera*. The book explained his theory that cholera was a water-borne disease. Still, despite the proof that Snow found on Broad Street, it took many years for the rest of the world to accept his views. Today, however, Snow is recognized as one of the first people to ever use meticulous observation and maps to understand how a disease is spread. Epidemiology owes much to Snow, as do the people whose lives his research has helped save.

Most scientists agree—the world is getting warmer. In recent years, studies have shown that temperatures around the planet are on the rise. In fact, according to the World Health Organization (WHO), 1998 was the warmest year ever recorded. And things are only getting hotter. The WHO estimates that the average temperature of the earth's surface will rise by 1.5 to 3.5 degrees Celsius (2.7 to 6.3 degrees Fahrenheit) by 2100.

If you like to go to the beach, this may come as good news. But global warming, as it's called, is not so simple. As the earth warms up, other environmental changes—some good, some bad—are likely to take place as well.

One environmental change that may take place thanks to global warming is a worldwide rise in the sea level. The WHO predicts that the sea level will rise by fifteen to ninety-five centimeters (six to thirty-seven inches) in the next 100 years. Why? One of the main reasons is something known as thermal expansion. As the oceans warm up, physical processes cause them to expand, or get bigger.

So what does this mean for cholera? Well, it's hard to know for sure, but some scientists believe that as the world's temperatures and sea levels rise, so will cholera outbreaks. One theory suggests that changes in ocean currents that result from thermal expansion will lead to upwellings along shorelines. Upwellings occur when an unusual amount of nutrient-rich waters, normally found near the ocean bottom, rise to the surface. For microscopic plants known as phyto-plankton, which float on the surface, drift with the currents, and thrive on such nutrients, upwellings mean feast time. Before long, the phytoplankton population explodes.

This population explosion triggers an interesting chain of events. When phytoplankton numbers increase, the typical result is a rise in phytoplankton-eating animals called zooplankton. And scientists have shown that cholera bacteria can live and multiply in the guts of certain kinds of zooplankton. In fact, one team of scientists believes that an increase in the zooplankton population may have been partially to blame for the 1991 cholera epidemic in Latin America that killed thousands of people.

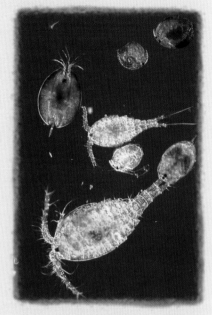

Zooplankton

Some scientists have serious problems with this global warming theory. They feel that the chance that global warming could lead to a rise in cholera epidemics is very remote. The reason they think this is because public health facilities are likely to improve over the years and should be efficient enough to counteract the effects, if any, of climate change; if the conditions for cholera do occur, doctors and others will be more able to cope with outbreaks. They also feel that recent cholera outbreaks have been due to poor public health measures—not ocean currents or phytoplankton blooms. Many of these same scientists think that more intensive research should be conducted before we jump to any conclusions.

4

CURRENT RESEARCH AND CURES

Cholera today has nowhere near the reputation it did a century ago. Whereas once it was a mystery, now scientists know almost everything that can be known about the disease. The goal now is not so much to learn more about cholera, but to cut the disease off at its source. By working to improve sanitation facilities around the world and by educating people on what they can do to avoid the disease, health activists hope to stop future outbreaks before they occur.

Staying Cholera-Free

Although cholera outbreaks continue to occur around the world, the chances of your contracting the disease are extremely low. In fact, according to the Centers for Disease Control, even if you're traveling in an area where cholera is common, your chances of getting the disease are about one in a million.

But even though the odds are in your favor, if you're traveling in an area with epidemic cholera, it is still wise to follow a few basic rules to ensure your health. The following is a list of things the World Health Organization recommends that you do (and don't do) when you're in a region where cholera may be present.

1. Drink only water that has been boiled or disinfected with chlorine, iodine, or other suitable products. Products for disinfecting water are generally available in pharmacies. Beverages such as hot tea or coffee, wine, beer, carbonated water or soft drinks, and bottled or packaged fruit juices are also usually safe to drink.

2. Avoid ice, unless you are sure that it is made from safe water.

3. Eat food that has been thoroughly cooked and is still hot when served. Cooked food that has been held at room temperature for several hours and served without being reheated can be a major source of infection.

4. Avoid raw seafood and other raw food, except fruits and vegetables that you have peeled or shelled yourself. Remember this simple rule: Cook it, peel it, or leave it.

5. Boil unpasteurized milk before drinking it.

6. Ice cream from unreliable sources is frequently contaminated and can cause illness. If in doubt, avoid it.

7. Be sure that meals bought from street vendors are thoroughly cooked in your presence and do not contain any uncooked foods.

Treating Cholera

Despite everything that can be done to avoid the disease, cholera still manages to strike many populations and kill thousands of people every year. Fortunately for those who do contract cholera, there are several things that can be done to keep the disease from becoming deadly.

The preferred method of treatment is very simple and usually successful. Since cholera victims die because of dehydration and complications that result from dehydration, the best thing to do is replace the fluids and salts lost through diarrhea and vomiting. Major aid organizations treat patients with a specially formulated oral rehydration solution, a prepackaged

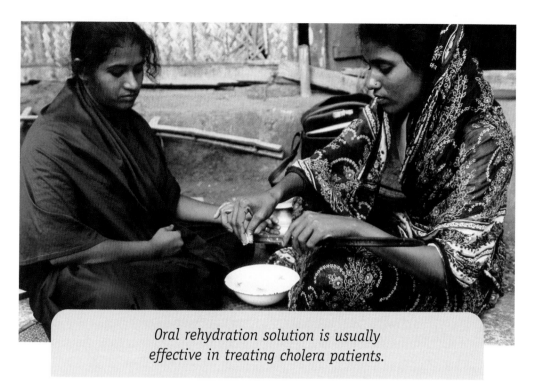

Oral rehydration solution is usually effective in treating cholera patients.

mix of sugar and salts that can be combined with water for easy drinking. This works almost 90 percent of the time. In exceptionally severe cases, however, when the patient is on the verge of death or is not able to drink the solution, doctors must force the fluids into the patient's body intravenously. In either case, less than one percent of patients die if they're able to rehydrate right away. On the other hand, case-fatality rates are as high as 50 percent when no treatment is available. This usually occurs in communities that are not prepared for a cholera epidemic and where there are no available facilities for treatment.

If you or your family are planning a trip to a country where cholera may be present, it's a good idea to do a little research before you go. Two organizations—the U.S. Centers for Disease Control (CDC) and the World Health Organization (WHO)—are great resources for cholera-related information. For up-to-date news on the latest outbreaks around the world, check out the Communicable Disease Surveillance and Response (CSR) division of the WHO Web site at www.who.int/emc/outbreak_news/disease_indices/ chol_index.html. If you're not on-line, contact WHO at its United States office, 525 23rd Street, NW, Washington, DC 20037; or call (202) 974-3000. Another option is to give the CDC's International Traveler's Information Line a ring. The number to call is (877) FYI-TRIP (394-8747). The Web site is www.cdc.gov/travel.

Some cholera patients are given antibiotics during the early stages of the illness. Effective antibiotics can help reduce the amount of diarrhea the victim has and the amount of fluids required for rehydration. For the patient, that's good news. The problem with antibiotics, however, is they don't do anything to stem the spread of cholera.

Vaccination

Researchers have developed both oral and injectable vaccines for cholera, but they're not particularly

"At present, the WHO has no information that food commercially imported from affected countries has been implicated in outbreaks of cholera in importing countries. The isolated cases of cholera that have been related to imported food have been associated with food which had been in the possession of individual travelers. Therefore, it may be concluded that food produced under good manufacturing practices poses only a negligible risk for cholera transmission."

—World Health Organization

effective because they only provide protection from the disease for a short period of time. The vaccine is made of dead *Vibrio cholerae* bacteria. The World Health Organization does not recommend it to travelers or to countries hoping to prevent the disease from crossing their borders. The WHO feels that vaccinations may give people a false sense of security and lead them to disregard other cholera-fighting measures that are much more permanent and effective, like stopping the disease at its source— usually the water supply. Likewise, international health regulations do not require any traveler to be vaccinated against the disease. That may change in the future, of course, as better, more permanent vaccines are developed. The Maryland-based National Institute of Allergy and Infectious Diseases (NIAID), a division of the U.S. government's National Institutes of Health (NIH), is currently testing new vaccines and new ways to treat cholera and other diarrheal diseases.

For the time being, the best cure for cholera is not a cure at all, but prevention. With a clean water supply, cholera has nowhere to go.

5

THE FUTURE

No one knows for sure what's in store for cholera in the near future. As the seventh pandemic continues to plague poor countries around the globe, health and medical experts keep doing what they can to treat victims and, most importantly, prevent outbreaks. Public health authorities in the United States and elsewhere are working to improve the ways they can predict where cholera will appear. They're also investigating new cholera outbreaks and educating the public about things that can be done to prevent the disease from attacking in the first place.

For now, residents of the United States face very little risk of contracting cholera, whether here at home or while traveling abroad. And as

If you like to eat, it's hard to argue: When it comes to versatility, the lowly, lumpy potato is hard to beat. Sure, it's just a dirty root. But pull it out of the earth and wash off the mud and there, in your hands, you'll find a world of edible potential. You can fry it. You can bake it. You can mash it. Chop it into chunks, slice it into slivers. Smear it with sour cream. The potato, without a doubt, has no culinary equal. Agreed?

It should come as no surprise, then, that scientists, working long hours, have discovered yet another possible use for the special spud. Using a relatively new scientific process known as genetic engineering, scientists have devised a way to make the potato work like a cholera vaccine. While in practice the process of turning a potato into an edible vaccine is very complicated, the idea itself is surprisingly simple: Take a microscopic sample of the cholera toxin and, using sophisticated laboratory techniques, insert it into a potato. Later, as the potato with this new gene grows, a tiny, safe-to-eat amount of the cholera toxin is present in every one of its cells. When a doctor then gives a bite-sized piece of the special potato to a patient to eat, the food acts exactly like a vaccination shot designed to increase the body's ability to protect against disease. As the potato is digested, the cholera toxin sticks like glue to cells in the patient's gut and causes the production of antibodies, which fight like fearless soldiers to destroy the toxin. Then, even after the toxin is defeated, the antibodies remain for months or even years, ready to do battle again if the need should arise. Should the patient run into real cholera during that time, whether because he or she drinks contaminated water or eats contaminated food, he or she is protected and won't get sick.

So, what does this mean for the world? For one, an edible vaccine would be nutritious. It would also be cheap. Potatoes, after all, are not exactly hard to come by. Finally, it's a lot easier to get people to eat potatoes than it is to convince them to get a shot. Still, there are potential drawbacks to genetically engineered potatoes. The main issue is that the environmental hazards of introducing strange genes into ordinary plants are not yet known. But another problem, at least as far as the potato is concerned, is that heat may make the medicine useless. For those who like their potatoes baked, this could prove difficult. The answer? Scientists are working on that one, but one solution is obvious: Instead of using potatoes, scientists could try using fruits or vegetables that people like to eat raw. Bananas anyone?

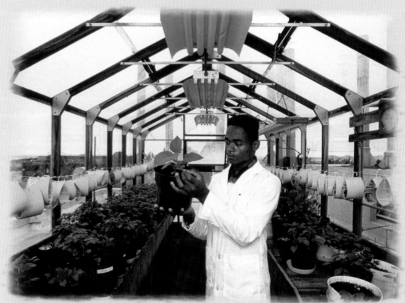

Scientists are using genetic engineering to make potatoes function as a cholera vaccine.

One of the interesting things about diseases like cholera is the fact that they often strike crowded, heavily populated areas—areas that may be too congested to maintain sanitary conditions. These places are often poor and lack basic health services. The people in such places may be more concerned with where they're going to find their next meal than whether they should wash their hands before they eat.

As the world's population grows, certain areas are becoming more and more crowded and diseases are becoming more and more common. Consider these statistics on population growth and ask yourself this difficult question: If the world's population continues to rise, yet the planet Earth remains the same size, where is everybody going to go? And how will they avoid the spread of deadly diseases?

- Worldwide, about 2.5 billion people were alive in 1950.
- More than six billion people were alive in 2000.
- The world population is currently increasing by about 70 million people per year.
- At the current rate of growth, the world population will hit seven billion by 2014.
- The population of India is expected to reach more than 1.2 billion by 2015.
- The population of Bangladesh is expected to hit 161.8 million by 2015.
- There were 270.3 million people living in the United States in 1998.
- The population of the United States will hit 304.9 million by 2015.

(All figures from the World Bank Group, www.worldbank.org)

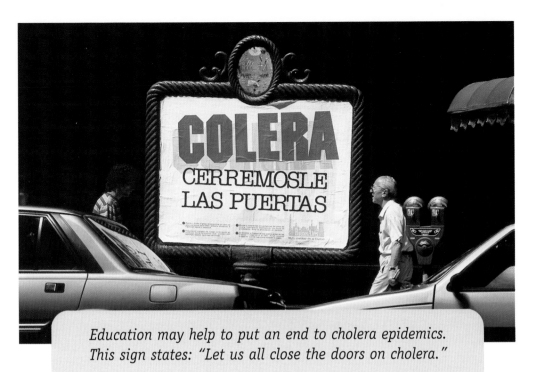

Education may help to put an end to cholera epidemics. This sign states: "Let us all close the doors on cholera."

health workers fight the disease in other parts of the world, the risk should decrease even further. Still, that doesn't mean cholera is no longer a threat. Many poor and developing countries need the medical assistance and training that nations like the United States can provide. Fortunately, as medical professionals conduct more research and learn more about diseases like cholera, they can better help the areas that need it most and develop more effective strategies of prevention.

What will it take to put an end to cholera epidemics? Some believe the answer lies in education. Others think it will take major changes in the world's economy—the kinds of changes that allow developing countries to catch up to the rest of the world and focus on food, water, and basic health measures rather than merely surviving. Still others see war as the problem because it brings so many people together in unsanitary and unhealthy conditions. In fact, cholera will never disappear from the planet until all of these problems are effectively dealt with. Someday, perhaps, the world will be rid of this deadly disease, but that day is not yet in sight.

GLOSSARY

antibiotic   A substance made by scientists, and given to infected patients, that kills or stops the growth of microorganisms that cause disease.

bacteria (bacterium)   Single-celled microscopic organisms that sometimes cause disease in humans, animals, or plants, but which are often harmless or beneficial to life.

case-fatality rate   The proportion of people with a particular disease who die because of it. For example, a case-fatality rate of 20 percent means that twenty out of every 100 people who acquired the disease died.

Centers for Disease Control and Prevention (CDC)   An agency of the United States government that works to improve health and quality of life by preventing and controlling diseases, injuries, and disabilities.

circulatory collapse A condition in the human body that occurs when the circulation system (heart, blood vessels, etc.) fails to work.

contaminate To make impure or unclean.

dehydrate To lose more body fluids than normal, whether because of vomiting, diarrhea, or other bodily problems. Severe dehydration can lead to death if left untreated.

disease A change in the normal structure or function of any part of the body, characterized by specific unpleasant symptoms or signs.

epidemic Also known as an "outbreak," the sudden increase in occurrence of a particular disease in a community or population.

epidemiology A branch of medical science that examines and tracks how diseases occur in populations.

infection The invasion of a host (a human being, for example) by a microorganism. Infections may eventually lead to disease.

mapping The scientific method of mapping out where people are who come down with a particular disease in an effort to understand how that disease spreads. Also called medical geography.

medical geography The scientific method of mapping out where people are who come down with a particular disease in an effort to understand how that disease spreads. Also called mapping.

microbe A microorganism.

microorganism An organism that can only be seen with the aid of a microscope.

organism An individual living plant, animal, or microorganism.

outbreak A sudden rise in the occurrence of a disease in a particular area or population.

pandemic An outbreak of a disease that occurs over a large area.

phytoplankton Plankton composed of plants. Sea phytoplankton, which varies in amount depending on conditions like light and temperature, is the main source of food, directly or indirectly, of all ocean organisms.

plankton Free-floating microorganisms found in water.

plankton bloom A dramatic increase in the amount of plankton in a particular area.

rehydrate To restore fluids to a dehydrated person.

sanitary Clean.

sanitation The act of making sanitary, or clean.

vaccine A preparation of living or dead microorganisms that is injected into an animal or human to produce or artificially increase immunity to a particular disease.

World Health Organization (WHO) An agency of the United Nations whose purpose it is to promote physical, mental, and social well-being in people around the world. The organization works to strengthen nations' health services and prevent and control diseases, among other things.

zooplankton Plankton composed of animals. These small floating or weakly swimming organisms drift with water currents in the ocean. Along with phytoplankton, zooplankton are the main source of food, directly or indirectly, for all ocean organisms.

FOR MORE INFORMATION

American Medical Association (AMA)
515 North State Street
Chicago, IL 60610
(312) 464-5000
Web site: http://www.ama-assn.org

The Centers for Disease Control and Prevention (CDC)
1600 Clifton Road
Atlanta, GA 30333
(800) 311-3435 or (404) 639-3311
Web site: http://www.cdc.gov

Doctors Without Borders
6 East 39th Street, 8th Floor
New York, NY 10016

(212) 679-6800
e-mail: doctors@newyork.msf.org
Web site: http://www.dwb.org

Environmental Protection Agency (EPA)
Ariel Rios Building
1200 Pennsylvania Avenue, NW
Washington, DC 20460-0003
(202) 260-2090
Web site: http://www.epa.gov

National Institute of Allergy and Infectious Diseases
NIAID Office of Communications and Public Liaison
31 Center Drive, Room 7A-50
Bethesda, MD 20892-2520
(301) 496-1884
Web site: http://www.niaid.nih.gov

National Science Foundation
4201 Wilson Boulevard
Arlington, VA 22230
(703) 292-5111
Web site: http://www.nsf.gov

University of California, Los Angeles (UCLA)
School of Public Health
Department of Epidemiology

Box 951772
Los Angeles, CA 90095-1772
(310) 825-8579
Web site: http://www.ph.ucla.edu/epi/snow.html

The World Health Organization (WHO)
Regional Office for the Americas
Pan American Health Organization
525 Twenty-third Street, NW
Washington, DC 20037
(202) 974-3000
Web sites: http://www.who.org
           http://www.paho.org

In Canada

Clinical Trial Research Center
Dalhousie University
Department of Pediatrics
Halifax, Nova Scotia B3H 3J5
(902) 428-8992
Web site: http://www.dal.ca/~ctrc

Population and Health Branch
Bureau of Infectious Diseases
Health Protection Branch
Health Canada

Tunney's Pasture
Ottawa, ON K1A 0L2
Postal Locator: 0603E1
Web site: http://www.hc-sc.gc.ca

Web Sites

Healthlink USA-Cholera Information Section
http://www.healthlinkusa.com/70.htm

Scientific American
http://www.scientificamerican.com

FOR FURTHER READING

Barua, Dhiman and William B. Greenough, III. *Cholera (Current Topics in Infectious Disease)*. New York: Plenum Publishing Corp., 1992.

De Castro, A. F. P., and W.F. Almeida, eds. *Cholera on the American Continents*. Washington, DC: International Life Sciences Institute Press, 1993.

Keusch, Gerald T. *Cytokines, Cholera, and the Gut*. Burke, VA: IOS Press, Inc., 1997.

Kudlick, Catherine J. *Cholera in Post-Revolutionary Paris: A Cultural History*. Berkeley, CA: University of California Press, 1996.

Kuwahara, S., and N.F. Pierce, eds. *Advances in Research on Cholera and Related Diarrheas*. Norwell, MA: Kluwer Academic Publishers, 1983.

Rosenberg, Charles E. *The Cholera Years: The United States in 1832, 1849, and 1866*. Chicago, IL: University of Chicago Press, 1987.

Snowden, Frank M. *Naples in the Time of Cholera, 1884–1911.* New York: Cambridge University Press, 1995.

Wachsmuth, I. Kaye, Paul A. Blake, and Ojan Olsvik, eds. *Vibrio Cholerae and Cholera: A New Perspective on a Resurgent Disease.* Washington, DC: ASM Press, 1994.

INDEX

CREDITS

About the Author

Chris Hayhurst is a freelance health and science writer living in northern Colorado.

Photo Credits

Design and Layout

Evelyn Horovicz